Together is better

Creating a community where each person belongs
A guide to fostering community inclusion for individuals with disabilities

Toni,
Keep your passion for community!

Written by
Al Condeluci, PhD, Kristen Burke, Melva Gooden-Ledbetter,
Mary Ann Evans McGuirk and Dori Ortman

Lash & Associates Publishing/Training Inc.

Library of Congress Control Number: 2007940681

Copyright © 2008 Lash & Associates Publishing/Training Inc.

All rights reserved. No part of this book may be reproduced, stored in a retrieval system, or transmitted in any form or by any means, electronic, mechanical, photocopying, recording, or otherwise, except for brief reviews, without the prior written permission of the publisher.

Published by Lash & Associates Publishing/Training Inc.
708 Young Forest Drive, Wake Forest, NC 27587
Tel: & Fax: (919) 562-0015

This book is part of a series on brain injury among children, adolescents and adults.
For a free catalog, contact Lash & Associates
Tel. & Fax (919) 562-0015 or visit our web site *www.lapublishing.com*

You may order this book directly from the publisher by calling (919) 562-0015 or visiting our web site www.lapublishing.com

Table of Contents

About the Authors..v

Acknowledgments..vii

Introduction: Beginning the Journey...1

Chapter One: Community and Social Capital...5
    Defining Community..9
    The Concept of Social Capital..11
    Creating a Sociogram..13
    The Theory of 150...16
    Building Tolerance...18
    The Process of Cultural Shifting..19

Chapter Two: What Makes Us Common..23
    Determine What Makes Us Common..23
    Implementing the Interest Profile..25
    Tying It All Together...26

Chapter Three: Finding the Community..29
    Find the Community Where the Passion is Regularly Celebrated....29

Chapter Four: Understanding the Community..35
    Understand How the Community Operates......................................35
    Activity Analysis...41
    Other Considerations..42

Chapter Five: Finding the Gatekeeper..45
    Find and Engage the Gatekeeper...45
    The Positive Gatekeeper...47
    The Gatekeeper..48
    Recruiting the Gatekeeper..49
    Toward Friendships...50

Conclusion: Journeying Forward...53
Appendices..57
Resources..75
Bibliography..76

About the Authors

Al Condeluci

Al has been an advocate and catalyst for building community in Western Pennsylvania since 1970 and currently serves as the CEO of United Cerebral Palsy (UCP) of Pittsburgh. He is a national leader and consultant on human services and community issues, speaking to some 15,000 people annually both nationally and internationally. He has authored many books, including *Cultural Shifting, Beyond Difference, Interdependence, The Essence of Interdependence* and *Advocacy for Change: A Manual for Action.*

Kristen Burke

Kristen is the project coordinator for UCP of Pittsburgh's Unique Community Partnership for Kids (UCP Kids) program. This allows her to support families in forming relationships in the community and to educate the community venue on the value of inclusion. Kristen is an Occupational Therapist and has worked for UCP of Pittsburgh for the past four years in a variety of roles.

Melva Gooden-Ledbetter

Melva is the Director of Centre Services at UCP of Pittsburgh. She has supported various disability populations for more than 20 years in the areas of residential, life skills education and vocational supports. She has co-authored articles appearing in the *Journal of Pediatric Rehabilitation* and the *Journal of Vocational Rehabilitation.*

Mary Ann Evans McGuirk

Mary Ann has spent the last thirteen years advocating for children with disabilities and is herself the mother of a child with special needs. She lectures at high schools and colleges, organizing and presenting school assemblies on disability awareness. She is the coordinator of the Family Advocacy Network and a Family Partner with UCP Kids, working with families of children with special needs to become involved in their communities.

Dori Ortman

Dori is the founder of CARE 21, an organization dedicated to building Community, Awareness, Resources, and Enrichment in the lives of families touched by Down syndrome. CARE 21 inspires families to help children reach their fullest potential, as Dori also strives to do with her own daughter with Down syndrome. Dori is also a Family Partner with UCP Kids, working with families of children with special needs supporting their inclusion in community recreational activities.

Al Condeluci, PhD
CEO - UCP of Pittsburgh
4638 Centre Avenue, Pittsburgh, PA 15213
412-246-2122 - 412-683-4160 fax
acondeluci@ucppittsburgh.org

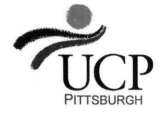

Acknowledgments

Together is Better is about change. It looks at how things have come to be, but more importantly, it is about how things can be *better*. It takes aspects of community and describes how those aspects can ebb or flow to enhance the lives of people. It builds on the simplicity of community, but understands the complexity that can sometimes come into play to make change happen.

This blend of simplicity and complexity is a good theme when acknowledging the creation of this type of manual. Books can be simple things – words on paper that build to concepts. But when applied, these concepts can help stimulate breathtaking and often complex change.

The same is true for our acknowledgments. In a simple manner, we must thank those people and groups who were instrumental in helping ***Together is Better*** unfold. Of course, the complexity is in recognizing that, with a manual of this type, where do you start?

First and foremost, we need to thank the great folks at the Heinz Endowment for their interest in this project and willingness to invest in the effort. Marge Petruska was the visionary who endorsed our idea and then Carmen Anderson helped make it happen.

Next we must thank all those associated with UCP/CLASS. This organization deals regularly in creativity, and the endorsement of the Board of Directors and key staff was integral to the development of this project. Board President Thomas Motley and staff members Dan Rossi and Joyce Redmerski were critical to this effort. Also thank you to the Family Advocacy Network, who served as our Advisory Board, and the families of CARE 21, in particular Vicki McGoey for her willingness to review ***Together is Better*** – not only with the eyes of a professional editor, but also from the viewpoint of dedicated mother to Joshua and Elena.

Of course, ***Together is Better*** could not have happened if not for the families that we support. Their passion, willingness and commitment to full community stand as a beacon for change.

Last we would like to thank our own families. Dan and Kailey Burke; Dave, David Evan, Lauren, Lindsay, and Nicole McGuirk; Brian, Joey, and Emily Ortman; Clyde and Lamar Ledbetter; and Liz, Dante, Gianna, and Santino Condeluci. Without their constant love and support, we could not have made ***Together is Better*** happen.

Al Condeluci, Kristen Burke, Melva Gooden-Ledbetter, Mary Ann McGuirk and Dori Ortman   Pittsburgh, PA   August 16, 2004

Introduction
Beginning the Journey

"Success is a journey, not a destination. The doing is often more important than the outcome."

~ Arthur Ashe

The young girl's love of dance started at around age 3. She saw a ballerina dancing on TV and thought that she was the most beautiful princess she ever saw. Her mom was thrilled that she took such an interest in dance, and they immediately went together to buy a ballerina bedspread for her room. Over the next couple of years, the girl continued to love watching ballerinas dance on TV and often told her mother that she was going to be a ballerina when she grew up.

Her parents took her to see The Nutcracker, and she sat glued to her seat watching the story unfold. Her mom bought her a ballerina outfit and she would gleefully wear it around the house, pretending that she was dancing on stage to the delight of the cheering audience.

When she was about 6 years old, her mother saw an advertisement in the local paper for a new dance class for 6 and 7 year olds. With much anticipation, the mother called the number to talk to the dance teacher. The teacher seemed very kind and was excited to be starting this new class. She said that quite a few children had already registered. Fearing that all of the spots would quickly fill, the mother didn't hesitate in signing her daughter up for the class, which started on the following Saturday.

Saturday morning, the little girl woke up early, filled with excitement about becoming a true ballerina. She insisted on wearing her ballerina costume and her mother told her that she looked like the most beautiful princess she ever saw. They drove to the dance class, both of them eagerly anticipating what was to come. But when they walked in the door, the dance teacher seemed to frown when she saw the little girl. She quietly pulled the mother aside and rebuked her for not indicating that her daughter had "problems." The teacher said this dance class wasn't for children "like her" and that she would be better off at a dance class especially for *"that type of child." The mother glanced over at her daughter, who still had a huge smile on her face and was already interacting with the other children. With tears welled up in her eyes, the mother wondered what was the easiest way to break her daughter's heart.*

A True Story

United Cerebral Palsy of Pittsburgh (UCP of Pittsburgh) through its Community Living and Support Services (CLASS) program provides services to individuals and families. Our mission is one of inclusion — *"working toward a community where each belongs."* We assist adults, and support their independence and community involvement, and our Unique Community Partnership for Kids (UCP Kids) program assists children with special needs in becoming involved in typical recreational activities. We created *Together is Better: Creating a Community Where Each Belongs* as a how-to guide for individuals and families to integrate into recreational activities and communities themselves, so that stories like the little girl who loved to dance never have to happen to another child.

The process of discovering how best to help someone become involved in a community is unique and is, in fact, a journey of discovery that is distinct for each individual.

While we take a direct look throughout the manual at how children and adults with disabilities can be integrated into community, please note that the concepts that we explore can relate to *any* individual, with or without a disability.

Just as individual personalities differ, so do abilities, talents, and interests. As such, the process of discovering how best to help someone become involved in a community is unique and is, in fact, a journey of discovery that is distinct for each individual.

Together is Better is our attempt to guide you through this journey, and it is intended to be interactive. Readers will note several written "exercises" throughout the manual and may wish to have additional paper on hand for extra writing space. We will also explain how to use the various forms included in the appendix. And, along the way, the narrative will teach you more about communities, how they interact, and how to best become a valued member of one.

Our vision for Together is Better is that it should prove useful for a variety of people. Parents might use this manual for their child with special needs, a professional will find it useful in helping a consumer, or an individual may wish to use the manual for his or her own journey.

Together Is Better is for persons of all abilities and ages. While we wished to make the narrative feel unique to each reader, it was impossible to consistently address each individual reader solely. As such, readers may find themselves reading a section that doesn't seem to apply to their needs. For instance, readers using the manual for an adult (either for self or for another adult) will find themselves reading sections pertaining to the interests of a child. In turn, parents using the manual for their child will read portions describing an adult activity.

Please be assured that *each section of the manual is equally important to all readers*. It is important to read the manual in a general context and to interpret and then apply each section, topic, and exercise to your unique situation.

> *Together is Better* set[s] the stage to adopt a process that will be helpful in relationship building and will help to seamlessly bridge a gap between people with disabilities and community.

While this manual does not guarantee full inclusion in every situation, it does set the stage to adopt a process that will be helpful in relationship building and will help to seamlessly bridge a gap between people with disabilities and community. Furthermore, it does not replace the natural role of the parent, family, or friend to assist a loved one with the process of developing relationships. It is hoped that this manual offers suggestions on how to enhance the process and encourage success.

It should further be recognized that every situation is unique and should be treated individually. The individual being supported may experience success in one venue and not in another, depending upon the culture of the community.

This should not be seen as a failure of the individual/family or even of the process, but may be related to the community's difficulty in accommodating the person seeking involvement in that community.

It is indeed a process — a journey ... perhaps for yourself, a loved one, a child, a client, or a friend. But be *certain* that it is a worthwhile journey.

"Believe something and the universe is on its way to being changed. Because you've changed, by believing. Once you've changed, other things start to follow."

~ Diane Duane

Chapter One
Community and Social Capital

"What we do in our lives individually is not what determines whether we are successful or not: what determines if we are a success is how we affect the lives of others."

~ Albert Switzer

Together is Better looks at a community approach that is rooted in the concept of interdependence and is a companion to the book *Cultural Shifting: Community Leadership and Change* (Condeluci, 2002). While *Cultural Shifting* provides an in-depth, comprehensive examination of interdependence, and we encourage you to read it to further grasp the notion of fully integrating oneself into a community, you need not have read *Cultural Shifting* to fully utilize the ideas presented in this guide. For purposes of this manual, an overview of the concept of interdependence is presented in preparation for setting the tone for the notion of "cultural shifting" and "finding the gatekeeper."

> **Interdependence:** Is defined as the relationship between two entities that assist someone to complete tasks that they are unable to do for themselves.

The concept of interdependence should be viewed as a positive step to encourage relationship building while allowing a person who is experiencing difference to accomplish those tasks that are challenging and still be an active part of his or her community.

> **Cultural Shifting:** A process that leads to a change within a community through the exploration of incorporating difference.

In *Cultural Shifting*, we explore the concepts of appreciation, acknowledgment, and acceptance as keys to community inclusion. To become more included, the concept of interdependence suggests that people with disabilities become involved in community, and as society learns about their common capacities and gifts, the value of these individuals begins to rise. Ultimately, acceptance within their communities occurs.

Finally, the concept looks at the commonality between people with and without disabilities. It is through these similarities that people find what they have in common and, thus, develop a conversation and begin to see each other in the same light despite their difference and/or diversity.

This approach of cultural shifting is designed to change societal perceptions of people with disabilities so that community is seen by all as a viable and natural option for people of difference. Past history (and still today) tells us that people with disabilities have been offset and often held to perceptions based on the Medical Model.

This model starts by:
- Articulating the person's deficits
- Labeling the person with a diagnosis or condition
- Addressing the "problem" with the professional being seen as the expert
- Suggesting that the person needs to be fixed and prescribing a treatment

The hope is that the person can be changed or treated to show normal behavior according to societal and professional standards and then be able to return to community.

The Interdependence Model, on the other hand, approaches this process from a capacity orientation. Rather than focus on the challenge, Interdependence suggests we look at the *capabilities* within the person with a disability. This Interdependence Model:
- Encourages relationship building
- Is driven by the consumer
- Promotes micro management (focuses on one's individual abilities)
- Promotes macro management (focuses on family, friends, and community)

The Interdependence Model promotes the idea that people with disabilities have the same desires, wants, and needs that any other person has and that people with disabilities have a choice in the decisions that they make.

A comparison of the Interdependence Model with the Medical Model is summarized as follows:

Interdependence Model	**Medical Model**
Focuses on capacities	Focuses on deficiencies
Stresses relationships	Stresses segregation
Driven by the consumer	Driven by the professional
Promotes micro/macro change	Promotes fixing consumer

While we realize that medical intervention is necessary for certain health aspects related to one's disability, the medical model should not carry over into the holistic view of the person. And it definitely will not promote cultural shifting. However, when necessary medical interventions are combined with the overall process of interdependence, it sets the stage for cultural shifting. It holds that when a new person enters the community, his/her presence is the catalyst for positively reshaping the culture. The following story illustrates the stark differences between the medical model and the interdependence model.

"In 1971, I had just graduated from college and was anxious to get started in the field of human services. I was fortunate to land a job as a medical social worker at a nearby hospital. I couldn't wait for my first day.

As I drove up to the hospital, I was struck by how large and imposing it was. I couldn't believe that close to 1,200 elders, with an average age of 87, lived in this facility. I was looking forward to doing the best I could.

As I walked into the hospital lobby, I noticed a young man, only a bit older than me, sitting in a wheelchair by the window. He saw me and raised his arm, calling me over to him. As I approached him, I noticed that he had a tray on his wheelchair with an alphabet board. He began pointing to the letters on the board and spelled out, "Hi, my name is David, do you work here?"

I introduced myself and told David that it was my first day of work at the hospital. David seemed to pause, and he looked intently at me. He then spelled out, "Get me out of here. I don't belong here."

Over the three years I worked at the hospital, I came to know David well. He was one of a few individuals with disabilities who lived at the hospital, amongst its hundreds of elderly patients, because, seemingly, there was nowhere else for him to go. David and I had many conversations during my years at the hospital. We were roughly the same age, and I greatly enjoyed spending time with him. He taught me many things about disability, about life, and about perseverance.

In 1973, I left the hospital to take a job with United Cerebral Palsy (UCP) and start my graduate studies at the University of Pittsburgh. The last thing I did when I left the hospital was make a promise to David that I would come back and get him out.

It took two years, but with support from UCP, we were able to help David move out of the hospital and into his own apartment. This was the start of a new life for him. When David lived at the hospital, he had always enjoyed listening to music.

When he began living in his apartment, he decided to join a local music club and began socialization with people his own age. He became an active and valuable member of his community."

Al Condeluci

Although this story took place many years ago, the realities of segregation still exist today. David was placed in an institution where the medical model felt he belonged. Today, children and adults with disabilities are segregated into special groups and activities where society feels they belong. As such, the medical model endures.

When the interdependence model was introduced, David's life improved dramatically by allowing him to form friendships with his peers based on similar interests. His community also benefited by embracing difference and welcoming a new member.

Together is Better is based on the concept of cultural shifting, and on the experiences of our organization, UCP/CLASS of Pittsburgh, and how we have implemented the steps of cultural shifting over the past several years. Taking the concept of interdependence, community inclusion and the role of the gatekeeper – an already existing group member who facilitates the acceptance of a new member – UCP/CLASS of Pittsburgh has developed model programs to demonstrate the techniques that are helpful to ensure the success of these concepts. We will describe the key steps in greater detail, as well as provide examples of how to implement these concepts.

Gatekeeper: An already existing group member who facilitates the acceptance of a new member.

In the many years that we have worked with individuals with disabilities or with families who have children with disabilities, we know that one of the greatest common concerns relates to finding friends and being active members of community. All parents want to see their children succeed, and we almost intuitively know that generally the greater number of friends they have and the stronger the relationships they are in, the greater the potential for success. Connections and belonging naturally reflect the health of the individual and the community. Certainly this is true for adults, as well.

Relationships and friends are the touchstone of a deep and rich life. *Together is Better* explores the notion of community and what it takes to begin the friendship process. We will look at formal definitions of community and trace back the initiation of friendship to the concept of "social capital." First, however, let's explore community.

Defining Community

Community: Is defined as *"a network of people who regularly come together for some common cause or celebration* (Condeluci, 2002)."

A community is not necessarily geographic, although geography can define certain communities. To come to an understanding of community is to appreciate that community is based on the relationships that form, not on the space utilized. In fact, space can be an abstract notion when it comes to understanding community. Think about the global community created by the Internet. These communities are not bound by geography, but rather are relationships forged in cyberspace.

The term "community" is the blending of the prefix "com," which means "with," and the root word, "unity," which means togetherness and connectedness. The notion of being "with unity" is a good way to think about the concept of community. When people come together for the sake of a unified position or theme, you have community.

Think now about communities in your life. All of us have a number of groups that meet the definition of community. Our families, for example, are a good framework for understanding community. These are people with whom we spend a great deal of time on common themes.

To help us just a bit more in understanding community, consider another definition of community from Robert Bellah (1985):

> *"A community is a group of people who are socially interdependent, who participate together in discussion and production, and who share certain practices that both define the community and are nurtured by it."*

Both of these definitions give us a solid start in thinking about communities in our lives.

Using the definitions of community, spend some time now identifying these groups in your life. List three communities you relate to on a regular basis.

1. _____
2. _____
3. _____

Often when you think about community, the notion of culture is introduced.

Culture: Is the learned and shared way that communities do particular things.

The term "culture" is dependent on community, as culture relates more to the behaviors manifested by the community. People bound together around a common cause create a community, and the minute they begin to establish behaviors around their common cause, they develop a culture. Culture is the learned and shared way that communities do particular things.

The three key features of community are:

1. Diversity of membership
2. Commonality of celebration
3. Regularity of gathering

This basic approach to community and culture blends three key features. One is the fact that community is a network of people and, often, these people may have great **differences or even distances (diversity)** between them. They can be different in age, background, ethnicity, religion, or many other ways, but in spite of their differences, their commonality or common cause pulls them together. The **similarity of the common cause or celebration (commonality)** is the second key feature of community and the glue that creates the network. Regardless of whom the members of the network are as people, their common cause overrides whatever differences they may have and creates a powerful connection.

Finally, as the collection of people continue to meet and celebrate **on a regular basis (regularity)** they begin to frame behaviors and patterns and become a culture, the third key ingredient. These regular meetings bond the community members as they discover other ways that they are similar.

The Concept of Social Capital

One of the most important facets of community is that it sets the stage for friendships and promotes the initiation of "social capital" for the members who belong.

> **Social capital:** Is another name for friendships and refers to the connections and relationships that develop around *community and the value these relationships hold for the members.*

Like physical capital (the tools used by communities), or human capital (the people power brought to a situation), "social capital" is the value brought on by the relationships.

L.J. Hanifan first introduced the idea of social capital in 1916. He defined it as:

> *"Those tangible substances that count for most in the daily lives of people: namely goodwill, fellowship, sympathy, and social intercourse among the individuals and families who make up a social unit… The individual is helpless socially, if left to himself… If he comes into contact with his neighbor, and they with other neighbors, there will be an accumulation of social capital, which may immediately satisfy his social needs and which may bear a social potentiality sufficient to the substantial improvement of living conditions in the whole community. The community as a whole will benefit by the cooperation of all its parts, while the individual will find in his associations the advantages of the help, the sympathy, and the fellowship of his neighbors."*

More recently, Robert Putnam (2000) defined the concept of social capital as:

> **"Referring** *to connections among individual's social networks and the norms of reciprocity and trustworthiness that arise from them…[It] is closely related to… civic… virtue… A society of many* **virtuous but isolated individuals is not necessarily rich in social capital."**

A key element then for social capital is the notion of **reciprocity**. This notion of doing things for one another is an important delineation between and among relationships. Quite simply, the reciprocal relationships in your life are the ones that keep you safe and fulfilled as a person.

Social Reciprocity: When friends help friends.

Think about the many communities with which you or your children are involved. People who might be different from you in many ways still surround you — your family, your work team, your church, your clubs or associations — but the commonality of these communities tends to override the differences you have with the other members and creates a strong norm for connections. Further, these relationships become helpful to you for social reasons. Sociologists call this helpfulness *"social reciprocity."* Quite simply, this is when friends help friends.

In a more global perspective, social capital is critical to a community because it:
- allows citizens to resolve collective problems more easily
- greases the wheels that allow communities to advance smoothly
- widens our awareness of the many ways we are linked
- lessens the tendency to fight or be aggressive
- increases tolerance
- enhances psychological processes and, as a result, biological processes

This last point prompts Putnam (2000) to assert:

> *"If you belong to no groups, but decide to join one, you cut your risk of dying over the* **next year in half!"**

This is an amazing quote because it underscores the fact that social capital breeds life. It actually helps us live longer.

The fact that social capital keeps us safe, sane, and secure cannot be understated. Most of us tend to think that institutions, organizations, or special programs are the key to safety. Places like hospitals or systems like law enforcement are thought to keep us safe, but the truth is that these systems are not the key to keeping us safe or healthy. Rather, it is the opportunity for relationships offered by a community, as well as the building of social capital and important friendships, that set the stage for our safety. Simply stated, the most important element in the safety and happiness of the person for whom you are utilizing *Together is*

Better is his/her circle of friends and the reciprocity they create. In fact, it has been suggested that social isolation, or the opposite of social capital, is responsible for as many deaths per year as is attributed to smoking (Putnam, 2000).

Creating a Sociogram

As we think about social capital in this manual, we want you now to look a little deeper. One way you can bring your social capital to life is to use a sociogram to review your relationships. A sociogram is a "social map" of the people in your life. It is also a helpful tool to visualize the importance of these relationships. Sociograms have been used by sociologists and anthropologists over the years to frame overall relationships (Schlien, 1997). The sociogram provides a visual interpretation of a person's social capital and relationship patterns from initial acquaintances to deeper, more intimate relationships. By using a sociogram, parents, advocates, and support professionals can come to see the existing social capital and also can track growth and development of relationships over a period of time. What follows is a further exploration of how we have been using sociograms in our work at UCP/CLASS.

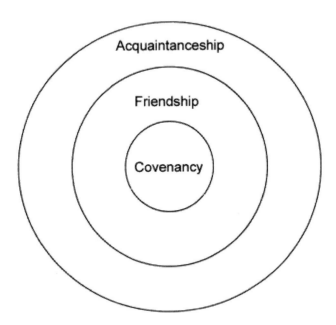

1. The Covenancy

In the space below, we want you to identify the first group of your sociogram, the people who are closest to you. Please write down the names of all those people in your life with whom you have a deep relationship. These are the people in your life that, if they left you, or were taken away from your life, you would be deeply wounded. These are the people you spend the most amount of time with and have the most reciprocity.

_____

_____

_____

_____

_____

Anthropologists call this listing of people our "sympathy" or "covenancy" group. These are the deepest and most important relationships in our lives. Of course, on this list are members of our family — wives, husbands, parents, children — the most intimate people in our lives. An interesting point with our "covenancy" group is that when you add up all the names in this category, most people average between 8 to 20 people.

This is interesting because, although we have the capacity to intimately love many people, we have finite constraints on our time. Consequently, we have only enough time to love (closely reciprocate) a handful of people.

2. The Friendship Zone

Moving on with our sociogram, we are now ready for the next group of people. In the space below, we would like you to identify all the people in your life with whom you regularly interact. These are the people with whom you share common interests and frequently engage in activities. In this group would be those people with whom you go to dinner, bowl, play bridge, go to the theatre, or whatever your mutual interests may be. These are your friends who are not merely casual friends, but friendships that manifest themselves, friends with whom you choose to spend quality time. Reflect a bit on this and then write their names below. Remember, these are people who often participate in activities with you but who are not included in your covenancy zone.

_____   _____
_____   _____
_____   _____
_____   _____
_____   _____
_____   _____
_____   _____
_____   _____
_____   _____

There are more lines for this group because there are usually more people in this category. These folks are ones with whom you share your time. You know more about this group because you see them in varying situations. In this category, even though we will all differ a bit, the usual range for most people here is between 20 to 60 people. Again, this listing can be limited because of the notion of time. You have only so many hours in a day to associate with people.

3. The Acquaintanceship Zone

Now to conclude the sociogram, we have the final category of people. We want you to identify all of the people who you know and even see regularly, but with whom you don't purposely engage in activities. These are acquaintances you have at work, church, and in the community. You know these people, but don't actually exchange any real time with them. In fact, this category often includes people from whom you purchase products or services in the course of your life. These people include your beautician or barber, the mechanic who fixes your car, medical personnel, or the butcher who cuts your meat. They might all be people you know, but never actually engage other than to buy what they offer. You see these people on a regular basis and know them, but aside from your purchase, you really don't interact with them. As you think about this list, name only the people who *currently* fit into this category in your life. We know that all of us have acquaintances from our past, but the people we want you to identify now are the ones in your life right now.

_____   _____
_____   _____
_____   _____
_____   _____

This group is often the largest in our sociogram, but it is our least reciprocal. Frequently the reciprocation is not much more than a wave, smile, or pleasantry. These people are certainly in your social capital range, but they are not the most important to your identity, safety, and security. Certainly, any of these individuals, over time, might move deeper into your sociogram. They are important candidates for reciprocity, but the most important people are in the first and second categories. If you venture to count the folks in this last group, research shows that the average ranges between 30 to 75 people.

The Theory of 150

As you step back from this exercise, there are some interesting reflections to consider. One is the total number of people in your life. When this type of exercise is done with large numbers of people, the total number of folks on sociograms is around 150 people. Some anthropologists feel that this is due to processes in the neocortex of the brain. One anthropologist by the name of Robin Dunbar has looked at neocortex size and the relationship to groups. Humans socialize in the largest groups of all primates. Dunbar feels that this is because we have the largest neocortex of all primates. In his work, Dunbar looked at social groups of primates in relationship to the size of their neocortex and found that Homo sapiens (humans) in this formula come out to 147.8. To this point, Dunbar says:

> *"The figure of 150 seems to represent the maximum number of individuals with whom we can have a genuinely social relationship, the kind of relationship that goes with knowing who they are and how they relate to us. Putting it another way, it's the number of people you would not feel embarrassed about joining uninvited for a drink if you happened to bump into them in a bar."*

Comparison of Relationships

The other interesting element of the sociogram is how the diversity fans out from the first group to the last. The people in our "covenancy" group are those most like us. The second group has a primary similarity to us, but also many differences from us. It is the differences these people display that really help us to grow. Think about any one person from your second list, the Friendship Zone. Extract that name in the space below and identify his/her similarities and differences from you:

Name

Similarities   **Differences**

_____   _____
_____   _____
_____   _____
_____   _____

As you look closely at how this person compares to you, we would contend that the similarities he or she has with you create a basic sense of security. The differences, however, are the things that cause you to grow. It is natural that this would happen, because the time you spend with this person, the commonality you share, is then tempered by the difference you have. The more "spicy" discussions you might have with this person, likely result through debate or discussions on your differences.

When we consider social capital for people with disabilities, we must recognize the void. Think of the person who you are trying to help and what his/her sociogram would look like. We have provided extra space in the appendix (Appendix A) for you to complete a sociogram for the individual for whom you are reading *Together is Better*. We know that children with disabilities still are separated from the greater community of kids and are mostly involved in special programs or services designed specifically for them. Adults with disabilities, too, are often relegated to separate support groups or gatherings with other people who have similar disabilities. In these realities, the major outlet for social capital is found only within the borders of the special programs. *To this extent then, the relationships that constitute the social capital of many children and adults with disabilities are other children or adults with disabilities. The narrowness of this reality leaves a significant void.*

This void leads to a couple of key challenges. One is simply the lesser number of people available for friendships. That is, if you are around only one kind of people, this then limits the number of friends you might find. The other challenge is found when diversity is limited. When people build friendships with people unlike them, the differences between them actually create personal growth.

Consider the notion of reciprocity. The more someone becomes connected with typical community, the more people begin to watch out for him/her. If one day a regular member of the group doesn't show up, a natural inclination would be for others to check up on him/her. This sense of group reciprocity is what leads to individual safety.

Another important aspect of reciprocity is that our differences actually fuel how reciprocity might unfold. That is, often when someone is reciprocal with us, they offer something we don't have or are not inclined to do for ourselves. For example, you might have a friend who helps you tune-up your car. His skill with machines may far exceed your ability. Conversely, you might have a talent for writing, so you help him with papers he needs to write in a graduate class he is taking. Our differences in skills are the basis for some of our reciprocity.

If the major social capital outlet for people with disabilities is other people with disabilities, then the reciprocity factor can become narrow. The narrower the confines of reciprocity, the less impact it offers.

Building Tolerance

Robert Putnam's ideas of how social capital builds tolerance and lessens pugnaciousness (the latent anger that can affect people) also fit closely to the concept of cultural shifting. Anthropologists have found that for communities to get better, new ideas, people, or products are necessary. By the same token, intolerant and angry communities are not as open or as ready to absorb new things.

Consequently, cultural shifting is more difficult when communities remain narrow. Social capital helps build tolerance because the exposure to others challenges us to consider new things. This developing openness then has an effect on pugnaciousness. Simply put, if you become more exposed to difference, anger levels have a greater potential to decrease.

This notion of social capital and the blending of similarity of interest with natural diversity of the members create a unique phenomenon for growth and development in both people and organizations. The drive to find, create, or be more than we were before is magically transformed when it is blended with community. The reciprocity developed through social capital is helpful, as well, for either specific or general reasons.

Cultures and communities have many features, but how social capital gets initiated and developed is tied to another one of the key ingredients of community — regularity. That is, for a community not only to be viable, but also to help people see beyond their differences, it must have some regular points of contact and connection. For a family community, this might be annual reunions or the celebration of holidays together. For a religious community, this would be weekly services and holy days for celebration. For organizations, this would be regular staff meetings or stakeholder gatherings. For clubs, groups, or associations, regular meetings or gatherings formalize the group as a community.

The more people come together, the more they find other ways that they are linked. That is, when a person first comes to a community he/she is drawn by the common interest of the community. As the individual attends again and again, he/she will find other similarities with people in the community and create a deeper sense of bonding.

Indeed, if we think about communities that we know, they all work toward some identified goal. From teaching people new skills, to saving souls, to addressing a common problem, to launching a government, all of these ventures capture the power of community, and then, through behavior, create a culture. The most vibrant and successful of these communities are the ones that have built more social capital.

The Process of Cultural Shifting

To promote the establishment of friendships and social capital requires not just an understanding of community, but also the ability to recognize the steps necessary to friendship. We call our process to build these steps to friendship "cultural shifting." As you will see in *Together is Better*, the four steps of cultural shifting are developed in later chapters, but we want to introduce them here. These steps are:

The four steps of cultural shifting:
1. Determine what makes us common.
2. Find the community where the passion is regularly celebrated.
3. Understand how the community operates.
4. Find and engage the gatekeeper.

Step 1 – Determine what makes us common.

This first step in the process of cultural shifting calls for the creation of an Interest Profile, which is further explored in Chapter Two. This profile is a listing of one's passions, hopes, dreams, skills, talents, capacities, and other positive elements of self. When you identify someone's passions, two very important things happen. First you set the tone for the person to feel empowered, important, relevant and unique. People love to talk about their passions and to feel validated when others want to know about them. The second key aspect is that the passions offer a ticket to the second step.

Step 2 – Find the community where the passion is regularly celebrated.

For every passion, it is our contention that a community exists somewhere. People gather around those things about which they feel good. Finding these gathering points is the critical challenge in this second step, which is explored in Chapter Three. Certainly, there are a number of ways to locate gathering points. We can look at the newspapers or local magazines, we can search the Internet, or we can simply ask people we know. Once we find the community, we are now ready to move on to the third step.

Step 3 – Understand how the community operates.

This step is about the infrastructure of community and is explored in Chapter Four. All communities, be they formal or informal, have rituals, patterns, jargon, and memory. The keys to success in the third step are to understand these things, become proficient in identifying them, and then coach the person you are helping to understand them. Once the community is understood, we are ready for the last step.

Step 4 – Find and engage the gatekeeper.

Every community has a myriad of members. Some of these members are influential with other members when it comes to new ideas. Further, some of these influential members, on some issues, show positive or negative tendencies. When a gatekeeper endorses or rejects a new person, often other people observing nearby will follow suit. In our way of thinking, these gatekeepers are the key to the acceptance (or rejection) of the person you are helping. Chapter Five explores how to find and engage gatekeepers.

And so, having had this opportunity to think about culture, community, and social capital, we are now ready to dig a bit deeper. Let's turn to the concept of finding community.

> *"You can learn more about a man in an hour of play than in a lifetime of conversation."*
>
> *~ Plato*

Chapter Two
What Makes Us Common

"I'd rather be failing at something I enjoy than be a success at something I hate."

~ George Burns

Determine What Makes Us Common

We've probably all heard it said that individuals with special needs are more like "typical" individuals than different from them. They have likes and dislikes, feelings and opinions. Certain things make them happy, while other things upset them. There are ways to motivate them and ways to calm them. These traits are true for *all* individuals. The first step in cultural shifting and helping an individual become involved in community is to find out what commonalities the individual has with the community. A great way to do this is to complete what we call an Interest Profile (a sample of an Interest Profile is included as Appendix B).

History and past treatment practices tell us that a variety of assessments are used to identify the needs of a person with a disability. However, more often than not, these practices have used the Medical Model, which leads to the assessments focusing on what the person *cannot* do. This further leads to the development of a goal plan and finally to a treatment approach to "fix" these things that the person cannot do. Interdependence, however, suggests another route — one that calls attention to the person's gifts and talents. To this extent, the Interest Profile serves as a means to get to know the person from a positive perspective, which then prepares us to locate community venues that positively relate to the person's interests. And it is in these venues that social capital can be found.

> **Interest Profile:** A means to get to know a person from a positive perspective and learn about his or her passions, hopes, dreams, skills, talents, capacities, and other positive elements of self.

You will note that the Interest Profile does act very much like an "assessment" inasmuch as it helps to narrow down specific traits about a person. However, because our focus is on the Interdependence Model and *not* the Medical Model, we don't even like to use the word "assessment." Therefore, we developed the user-friendly Interest Profile for our use in the UCP Kids program (see Appendix B), and it has been very effective. It offers parents and caregivers the opportunity to reflect upon their children's interests, needs, and competencies, so that children can be suitably matched to successful, fun, and fulfilling activities. The Interest Profile provided in Appendix B can be modified to determine the interests of adults and for individuals to reflect upon their own needs and interests.

Keep in mind that it is important to view the Interest Profile as a "stepping stone" in the journey of discovering how best to help someone become involved in community. It is a tool to be used *throughout* the process and will grow and change as new information unfolds.

The first step in conducting an Interest Profile is simply getting to know more about the person. In this step, we are looking to learn who the person is, what he/she likes and dislikes, and what some of the person's true passions might be. This involves spending time with the person and his/her family to become familiar with the individual's background, experiences, and strengths. The Interest Profile will also glean information about the person's current relationships/friendships, interests, personality traits, and methods of communication. You will also gather information on the types of activities in which the individual might wish to participate in the future.

You should begin this initial phase of learning more about the individual in an environment that is familiar and comfortable to him/her. If you are working with a child, the child's mother and/or father might introduce you if you have not previously met. Start by explaining what you are hoping to do and use easy small talk to engage in conversation. You might initiate conversation about school, friends, or something that the child likes to do. Take about 10 – 15 minutes just spending time with the child. For younger children, you may want to engage them in a more playful activity or a coloring activity to help set the tone. In working with adults, you should engage them in general conversation, while at the same time learning answers to the questions on the Interest Profile. In other words, and this is extremely important to keep in mind at all times, *the Interest Profile is a tool to help you gather information, but should not be used as a direct question and answer interview.* Discussions should be casual and friendly. Keep in mind to treat an adult with a disability with dignity and respect. Be concrete with your questions, but not patronizing.

Implementing the Interest Profile

You will note in the sample Interest Profile provided as Appendix B that there are both general questions and specific questions. There are also rating scales pertaining to group/activity participation and relationships. All of these areas are crucial in identifying how best to help the person become involved in community. By having a clear understanding of the relationships and the types of activities in which the person is currently vested, you will better be able to match the person into a new community.

At all times, you should remember that this is a *conversation* to discover an area of interest. It is imperative to remain focused on the person to best discover passions. If the individual has difficulty answering any of the questions, you should ask the question in a different way. You should also feel comfortable using open-ended questions that can lead to additional information or discussions about the person's interests. As the person is engaged in sharing information, you may find that you are learning answers to additional questions that occur later in the Interest Profile. You will gain a sense of how to engage the person, as well as his/her ability to communicate, maintain conversations, and interact with people. These, too, are important pieces of information that will be helpful when introducing the individual into a new community venue.

The Group and Activity Participation section of our sample Interest Profile categorizes questions in the following way:

- activities in which the family participates
- groups the person belongs to individually
- activities the person enjoys with other families or relatives
- neighborhood and community events the family attends
- school events (if applicable)

The most important component of this portion of the Interest Profile is the rating scale, with each activity rated as 1-Very Comfortable, 2-Somewhat Comfortable, 3-Uncomfortable or 4-Very Uncomfortable. Dependent upon where on this scale the person rates each of the questions, you should begin to gain a sense of the types of situations in which the person is most happy and at ease and, accordingly, what might ultimately be some true areas of interest.

Another area to consider when completing the Interest Profile is the comfort level of the individual's family in supporting his/her involvement in the community and activities of interest. When any new person enters into a group, there is an element of risk that they might not necessarily fit in or be successful in the activity initially. There is a natural adjustment period for any individual entering a new group, as well as an adjustment for the person's family and loved ones. Some questions to consider include:

- Will the family allow their loved one to take this safe risk?
- Will the family be willing to support the individual as they begin to learn about his or her group/community?
- How much, if any, involvement should the family have in the initial introduction of the group/community?
- When should the family pull back to allow their loved one some autonomy in the newgroup/community?

These are key questions, especially when working with children. This might be difficult for many families, particularly if their experiences have not been very positive in relation to past community involvement.

Tying It All Together

Once the Interest Profile is completed, you will have a better understanding of the individual with whom you are working. Now it's time to put it all together, decide on an area of interest and, ultimately, find community experiences that match that interest. You may wish to ask the individual's family to help you brainstorm ideas for possible community connections.

The key here is to be *creative*, at all times keeping in mind what the person **likes** to do, NOT only what the person **can** do. Here's when you need to think "outside the box." For instance, consider John's story. John was a truck driver who, after an accident, could no longer walk and would never be able to drive a truck again. John loved truck driving, and he often talked about driving a truck again. It was decided to try and find another community activity in which John could get involved. After completing an in-depth Interest Profile to discover John's interests, it was apparent that John's true passion was … truck driving! But John could never drive a truck again, so what activity could he possibly become involved in relating to truck driving? Here is what the person working with John creatively came up with: Once a week, John calls for an accessible van to take him to the local "truck stop." He goes in, hangs out with the truckers, discusses trucks, talks about where the truckers have been and where they're going, shares his own stories of trucking, and is very satisfied. John is well liked, the "regulars" all know him and look forward to seeing him when stopping at that particular hangout, and John is a true part of their community. And, most importantly, John is experiencing his true passion, and it is still an important part of his life.

So, again, discovering one's passion is not necessarily limited to what the individual *can* do … it is about what his/her interests truly are. John's story is an example of how a person's passion seemed unrealistic and out of reach. But by taking it and thinking of ways it can be extended in a broader sense, John was able to find a world where he is relevant and connects to people through sharing his passion, thereby building social capital.

In our UCP Kids program, we've often had to take a child's interest and passion and find ways to connect the child's dreams to what's going on in the "real world." One boy who dreams of becoming an astronaut, even though this is not possible because of his disability, is thrilled to now belong to a Star Trek enthusiasts club. He loves getting together with the other members to discuss space and the adventures of the Star Trek crew, and connecting with other people who share his passion. Another boy we worked with, who uses a wheelchair, had a passion for basketball. You'll read his story in Chapter Three and find out how he is now a valued member of a basketball team. The bottom line is that, while you do have to consider what is possible depending on an individual's abilities and talents, it is more important not to rule *anything* out.

Once you discover what a person's true passion is, the next step is finding a community venue that matches it. Chapter Three will explain in more detail how to locate and approach a community.

"If bread is the necessity of life, recreation is a close second."

~ Edward Bellamy

Chapter Three
Finding the Community

"Recreation offers the discovery of self satisfying pleasures... a time for social expression and much needed family cohesion."

~ Nancy M. Morrow

Find the Community where the Passion is Regularly Celebrated

In Chapter Two, we looked at the creation of an Interest Profile; that is, identifying one's passions, hopes, and skills. Also, before choosing a leisure activity, it is essential to identify the individual's present recreational patterns and competencies, as well as the interests of the individual and his/her family. What we learn through this process helps us to better find a suitable match for a successful and fun activity. For example, if an individual likes to dance, but has some issues with coordination, it might be better to find a creative movement class rather than tap or ballet. By taking part in a leisure activity, it gives people the opportunity to have fun together, meet new people, make friends, and experience a sense of belonging. Therefore, finding the setting where one will be accepted sets the stage for inclusion and cultural shifting.

It is important to note here that when we talk about community, we mean typical, generic community. There is no question that the trends today are to find separate or special communities for people with disabilities. Over and over, we know of situations where families of individuals with disabilities are turned away from typical community resources and directed to a special program for people with disabilities, such as the story of the little ballerina in the Introduction to *Together is Better*.

In fact, many families now think that these special places are the only places for their loved ones in a community. This is true for adults as well as children. There is a great hesitancy to accept an adult with a disability into typical groups because of fears and misunderstandings.

What has also fueled this reality are well meaning, but misguided human service agencies themselves. It is standard procedure for many agencies that serve children as well as adults with disabilities to set up special recreation, interest, or social groups. In some ways, these agencies and the human service system at large have created a "dualistic society."

When we think about these separate communities and this "dualistic society," it is easy to understand how this has happened. One key manifestation of the Medical Model is to congregate people who are different and to create treatment plans. The creation of segregated recreation or social groups for children and adults with disabilities is a type of specialized treatment. However, the blunt reality is that the longer we keep people with disabilities separated from typical community opportunities, no matter how noble the effort, the more we perpetuate the misunderstandings, stereotypes, and stigmas that difference can bring.

In a cultural shifting approach, you need to have a general understanding of the neighborhood in which you are identifying community activities. Resources in the vicinity need to be identified or developed, and efforts need to be made to ensure that the connection and progress are maintained. A community is not only a place where one lives or plays, but it is also a place where one feels connected.

This effort of linking people with disabilities to natural community activities is what we call "Community Building." Not only does this effort benefit the person with a disability, but it also improves overall community life.

Questions one should ask when analyzing a target area are:
- What are the strengths and challenges the vicinity has faced?
- What is the current population of adults and/or children?
- What are the economic conditions/employment rate? (This is not necessarily related to overall well-being; money and education do not mean that the area is strong.)
- Type of area (urban, rural, suburban)
- Social conditions? Do people know each other/what clubs or activities do children and adults participate in?
- Is it diverse?

After gathering this data, one can begin to develop a better understanding of what the target area has to offer. We call this effort "Community Mapping." Just as the Interest Profile discussed in Chapter Two "maps" the individual, so too must we understand the community.

The next step in this process is accumulating resources related to the target area and making them available to the adults and children with disabilities and their families. This can be a tedious process but critical to the potential success of the effort.

In order to help individuals become involved in typical community activities, one must be aware of what opportunities or possible opportunities exist within the neighborhood *and community* (Center on Human Policy, 1990; Center for Urban Affairs and Policy Research, 1998). This involves:

- Finding out about the use of various neighborhood and community places (who uses them, when, for what purpose).
- Finding out about local organizations and associations (where and when do they meet, memberships, etc.).
- Finding out where people go and what children/adults do who are of various ages, genders, religious affiliations, share similar interests, and so forth.

Below are some examples of local associations, institutions, and key informants that are possible community resources:

- Religious (church groups)
- Arts organizations (dance, crafts, theatre)
- Youth groups (YMCA, neighborhood centers)
- Parks and recreation departments
- Community associations (library, hospital)
- Schools (PTA, clubs, teachers)
- Health and fitness groups
- Sports leagues
- Service clubs (Lions, Rotary, etc.)
- Colleges/universities (utilize therapeutic recreation students to volunteer)
- Realtors (some have a list of activities or organizations that they present to prospective buyers)
- Local residents (parents) who have children in activities
- Community papers, bulletin boards, phone books

It is important to research these venues and find out what they have to offer. For instance, one may want to know if a church/place of worship has CCD programs, Sunday School, Vacation Bible School, choirs, or outreach groups. Are there volunteer opportunities as well as classes at the local library? Are there walking/running groups at the local fitness club? What sports leagues are not competitive — do all children participate at least some of the time?

It is also crucial when looking for resources to identify the logistics and distances. How far will the person travel for an activity? Does he/she have transportation? Who is responsible for program implementation? Do participants need to buy equipment, such as pads or helmets? Is there a cost? Is the facility accessible? Is the program designed to include everyone and can modifications be made? Planning and coordination of all details need to be researched and finalized before the individual begins the activity.

Community Mapping can help to find a leisure activity for an individual. David is an 11- year-old boy who loved the game of basketball, but because of his physical and cognitive disabilities, assumed he would never be able to participate on a team. He enjoyed playing his video games and watching basketball on television, and he understood the basic rules of the game. Therefore, it made sense to find an activity that somehow related to basketball.

David attended a specialized school, but the school did not have a basketball program. So we called the public school in David's neighborhood and talked to the athletic director, coach, and principal. After two months of calling back and forth and changing plan after plan, we knew we had to look elsewhere to find David an activity related to basketball. As we have mentioned, helping individuals participate in community activities can be an involved process.

We began investigating what else David's neighborhood had to offer. Where did the children gather to play ball? These were questions that led us in the direction of a local "Boys & Girls Club." We called and spoke with the director, who reiterated that "there are special programs for kids like David." We knew we weren't getting anywhere on the phone, so we asked for ten minutes of his time. He agreed to meet with us, at which time we explained the philosophy of our UCP Kids program. We also stressed the fact that David should not be penalized for his *disabilities*, but perhaps the program could be adapted so that he could use his *abilities*. David just wanted an opportunity to participate in "fun activities" with his peers. The recreation director then asked to talk to David and his family and offered to take them on a tour of the facility.

The following week, David, his mom, and a support person walked into a busy, loud recreation center. David felt overwhelmed and nervous from the noise and activity. His mom pushed him in his wheelchair, stopping to massage his arm and offer soothing words of comfort as they moved towards the gymnasium. The receptionist smiled and welcomed them and introduced them to the staff. The director talked with David and his mom, showed them around, and reassured David that he would soon feel at ease. He invited David to meet the players on the team and told him not to worry.

The recreation director took the time to get to know David and his mother. He offered to provide individualized support, as well as presented opportunities for the other members to interact with David. David became the team manager/scorekeeper, and sat on the bench with the team. He is now **one of the guys.** He had a role to fill — one that matched his interest.

The season lasted six weeks. At the last game, David received a shirt and a trophy. He cried tears of joy when the team invited him onto the floor to be recognized. The director encouraged David to come back.

David's teammates and staff learned that everyone can be part of a team, even if they do not have fully developed skills. Hence, this experience was not only beneficial to David and his family, but also to the staff and members of the club. The most important factor for an inclusive leisure activity to be successful and rewarding is the commitment of the staff to do whatever it takes to make it work.

Some factors to keep in mind:
- Be objective—do not say, "This cannot work here." Instead say, "How can we make it work?"
- If you encounter someone who says, "Special needs children/adults have their own groups," listen to what they have to say and let it be the beginning of the road, not a dead-end. Many people do not understand why people with disabilities need to be included.
- Describe the person in a positive way, so as not to focus on his/her needs and deficits.
- Try different strategies — stay flexible enough to abandon what does not work and go in another direction. Dig deep to find more resources; what might not work for one person could work for another.
- Find an activity that matches the interest or positive aspects of the individual. The activity should provide for building on existing interests and learning new abilities. Programs should also be age-appropriate.

- Observe the activities. Talk to an instructor or leader. Are there available supports?
- Understand the limits. Be realistic and do not rush to get results — adjust expectations.
- Some programs can be flexible enough to allow individuals to participate at their own pace, yet offer opportunities to improve over time (i.e. bowling, art, music, creative dance).

People with disabilities and their families want to become connected, but often they do not know how or where to start. Time is needed to create visions — building social capital does not happen quickly. A community must have a shared vision to incorporate diversity when welcoming new members. It is important to emphasize that inclusion benefits *all* people, not only those with disabilities. In the next chapter we will examine the elements of a community in order to determine the best way to facilitate a new member's acceptance.

"You can't hit a home run unless you step up to the plate. You can't catch fish unless you put your line in the water. You can't reach your goals if you don't try."

~ Kathy Seligman

Chapter Four
Understanding the Community

"Leisure/recreation is a state of mind. It is an inner place of peace and a **bridge** *which connects to others in a meaningful way."*

~ Kathy O'Kefee

Understand How the Community Operates

Community was previously defined as a network of people who regularly come together for some common cause or celebration. Step three in the process of cultural shifting is understanding the elements of a community. It is important to understand a community and the actions of its culture in order to be accepted into that community.

Community: Is defined as a network of people who regularly come together for some common cause or celebration.

Once a community has been identified, the best way to understand it is by observing the community in action and by talking to the people involved. By observing a group prior to participation, you are able to prepare and problem-solve ahead of time in order to avoid encountering problems once the person with a disability becomes involved with the activity. All communities have four common themes: rituals, social patterns, language or jargon, and history or memory. By observing a community and defining the actions in terms of rituals, patterns, jargon, and memory, it gives the newcomer clear thoughts that can assist in the process of joining.

The more we understand about these elements, the more likely we are to be accepted as part of that community

~ Al Condeluci, 2002

In order to gain a better understanding of the four key elements of any community, let's discuss these elements in a little more detail. As you read through this, think about the culture of the communities in which you participate.

The Four Elements of Community:
1. Ritual
2. Social Patterns
3. Language or Jargon
4. History or Memory

Rituals: A ritual is a deep-rooted behavior that the community holds as important. Some examples of common rituals are: a cheer that a team chants before a game to get the players pumped up and to promote team cohesiveness, a prayer at the end of a youth group, or a song at the end of a camping trip. Knowing and performing the rituals that a community holds as important is critical to becoming a valued member of that group. Every culture has rituals that center around whatever it is they are celebrating. It is essential to assist the person who you are trying to assimilate into a group in learning that group's rituals.

Social Patterns: The patterns of a culture refer to the movements and territory of the group members. Observing the patterns of a group can give information about how members relate to one another. This type of information becomes important when trying to identify gatekeepers and other critical connectors. Members of a group who meet on a regular basis often position themselves in the same area. Think about the places that you go on a regular basis, perhaps church, for example. Most people typically sit in the same spot each time. Patterning also refers to the location of the meeting. Changing the location of a meeting can affect how people relate to one another. If you take a group that typically meets in a classroom setting and move them to a park, the dynamic of the group will change.

Language or Jargon: Jargon refers to the words or phrases the culture uses to discuss, debate, or celebrate a common theme. An example of a time when learning the jargon of a group was critical was when UCP Kids assisted a child with becoming a member of a karate class. The instructor used Japanese terms throughout the class to describe the movements. The child who was joining the class had a language delay so that posed a challenge. It was important to work with this child to help him learn the different terminology. We obtained a list of the Japanese terms from the instructor and practiced them with the child ahead of time. We also taught the instructor how to best communicate with the child.

History or Memory: Memory is the history or legacy of a community and is another important dimension of a culture. Memory can include stories, photos, or folklore of the common theme of the culture. Cultures keep track of their history in many different ways. Some examples are through yearbooks, annual reports, and newsletters that weave the elements of community.

Think about the three communities that you listed earlier in Chapter One. On the following page, pick one of these three communities and identify the rituals, patterns, jargon, and memory that are a part of that culture.

Key Rituals:
_____
_____

How Do People Gather:
_____
_____

Unique Words:
_____
_____

Background of the Community:
_____
_____

Once you have answered these questions, think about how a person with a disability can fit into that group's culture. Will he/she require extra practice or adaptations in order to participate? Once you have observed and analyzed a community, you should have an understanding of the types of activities that the members of the community are expected to perform. When you consider all of the physical and cognitive components of the activity, you may think to yourself, "How will someone with a disability be able to participate in this activity?" The key to adapting any activity is to be creative and open-minded.

"We need to realize that different is not always wrong or ineffective but just a different way to approach a situation. We all adjust the things that we do to accommodate the situation that we are in presently".

~ Conroy

The way to adapt an activity will be unique based on the person's needs and the requirements of the activity, but following are some ideas to keep in mind.

Modify the Equipment

"Manufactured equipment is available through a number of adaptive equipment catalogues. However, since each individual has different needs, unique modifications will often need to be developed. Have ace bandages, easy-off adhesive tape, and duct tape on hand" (American Association for Active Lifestyles and Fitness). The following are some additional ideas for modifying equipment (American Association for Lifestyles and Fitness):

- Larger, lighter, slower moving balls
- Paddles/rackets with a larger contact area
- Brighter equipment to make tracking easier
- Build up handles with foam or tape to make them easier to grasp
- Equipment with handles can be shortened/lengthened

Be Creative!

Provide Structure and Routine

Individuals who happen to have disabilities (especially those with cognitive disabilities) tend to have a more positive experience when they are able to anticipate what is going to happen (Coyne, Nyberg, & Vandenburg, 1999).

Develop a checklist that will assist the individual in preparing for the activity. It should include information such as:

- Time and place
- Spending money (if needed)
- Transportation information
- Things to bring
- What to wear

(Coyne, Nyberg, Vandenberg, 1999)

Develop an activity card. Activity cards provide written and pictorial information about an activity. They are useful in preparing an individual for what will happen and in helping him or her to sequence the events of an activity (Coyne, Nyberg, Vandenburg, 1999). An activity card can be developed based on the individual's needs, but often includes information such as:
- Schedule
- Instructions
- Materials
- Rules
- People involved in the activity

(Coyne, Nyberg, Vandenberg, 1999)

Eliminate Distractions
- Keep background noise to a minimum
- Remove unnecessary equipment
- Play indoors during the learning phase
- Make sure the instructor(s) place themselves where they can be seen
- Keep equipment in the same place
- Try to avoid frequent changes in routine

(American Association for Lifestyles and Fitness)

Use Multiple Senses
- Use a variety of sounds and textures
- Verbally explain as well as demonstrate instructions – keep instructions simple!
- Hang pictures of a person performing the step of an activity

(American Association for Lifestyles and Fitness)

Manipulate the Environment
- Make the spaces smaller (shorten bases, use half the field)
- Use lines on the floor to instruct the person where to run
- Use brightly colored tape to identify boundaries and landmarks

(American Association of Lifestyles and Fitness)

Don't be afraid to change the rules!

Other important things to consider when observing a community are (Coyne, Nyberg, Vandenberg, 1999):

Dates and Times — It is important that the activity is held at a time that fits well into the person's schedule. If the person with a disability has to frequently miss an activity because of scheduling conflicts, he/she will not be given the opportunity to interact with other group members on a regular basis. When thinking about the time to schedule an activity, think about what is the best time of day for that person. For instance, scheduling an activity at a time when that person is usually sleepy may not be a good idea.

Costs — Whether or not someone can afford to pay for admission and equipment needed for an activity is a factor to consider when deciding upon an activity. If costs are an issue, one option is discussing a payment plan with the facility. Another option to consider (especially if the person requires an expensive piece of equipment) is approaching local community service organizations with a fundraising project.

Transportation issues — Does this person have a reliable source of transportation to and from an activity? Consider that he/she may need training in order to make access arrangements or learn a bus route if he/she does not have a vehicle.

Accessibility — It is, of course, important to consider accessibility when choosing an activity. People with disabilities have unique requirements based on their individual needs, but some basic things to consider when thinking about accessibility are: accessible routes of travel, adequate space, ramps, elevators, lifts, wide entrances, and accessible bathrooms. A good resource to have when considering accessibility is the Americans with Disabilities Act Accessibility Guidelines, which can be viewed on the ADA website at www.ada.gov.

Clothing and Equipment — We have already mentioned that it is important to think about the cost of clothing and equipment. If a person has difficulty dressing himself or herself, it is important to think about that ahead of time. Some solutions to this problem may be: dressing prior to coming to the activity; wearing clothes that are easier to put on and take off (no buttons or zippers, no tight clothing); providing someone to assist that person with dressing.

Is the Activity Age Appropriate? — It is more important for an activity to match the age of the individual rather than his/her skill level. Interacting with peers of the same age is the most important goal when participating in leisure activities.

It is essential to determine ahead of time whether the person with a disability will be successful in the activity/group. To do this, it is important to identify the person's specific needs and the specific skills that the activity requires. A useful tool to use when doing this is an Activity Analysis. An Activity Analysis requires you to break down an activity into steps, which makes it easier to identify specific obstacles.

The following is an example of an Activity Analysis (Schlein, 1997). All communities have activities that are performed on a regular basis; therefore this tool may be used in any community. When observing a group/activity, use the first column to write down the specific steps of that activity. If the person wishing to participate in the activity is able to complete that step of the activity independently, place a plus sign (+) in the middle column. If you feel that he/she will need assistance with that step, place a minus sign (-) in the middle column. For those steps with a minus sign in the middle column, use the last column to generate ideas about the types of adaptations or modifications that you could use.

The following example was completed while observing a karate class. The first column lists the steps of the karate class. Take a look at step two — "take off shoes." Notice that the minus indicates that the child was probably going to have a problem taking off his shoes. You will note in the last column that the adaptation we made to help the child complete this step of the activity was to wear shoes with Velcro so that he would have an easier time putting on and taking off his shoes. The Activity Analysis can be a helpful tool to use when preparing to join a group. Two blank Activity Analysis forms are included as Appendix C for you to use when making your own observations.

Activity Analysis
Karate Example

Steps of the Activity		Adaptations/Modifications
Enter gym		
Take off shoes		Takes increased time to take shoes off
Place shoes and bag in the corner		Wear shoes with Velcro

Together is Better

Greet instructor and other students	
Line up in straight line	Will learn through role modeling of peers
Warm-up / stretch exercises	
Listen to and follow directions from instructor	Instructor will demonstrate in addition to verbal instructions
Listen to the history of Martial Arts and learn some Japanese terminology.	May have difficulty understanding Instructor will modify as needed
Set up obstacle course (hoops, mats, cones)	Demonstration
Perform obstacle course (run, jump, strike)	Demonstration
Learn strikes hands and feet (verbal directions and demonstration)	
Learn positions (stand, sit, kneel) (verbal directions and demonstration)	
Learn breathing techniques (verbal directions)	May require modification and increased repetition
Break to drink from water fountain	
Cool down	
Review skills and outline tomorrow's activities	Simple verbal directions

Other Considerations

The following are characteristic of activities that typically allow for greater success (Coyne, Nyberg, Vandenberg, 1999):

Be age-appropriate — It is more important for the activity to include peers of the same age rather than peers of the same ability. Being around peers of the same age increases the opportunity for socialization and creating friendships.

Be of interest to the person — This may seem fairly obvious, but it can often be overlooked if the activity that is of interest to the person with a disability seems too challenging. Think back to the story about David who uses a wheelchair and wanted to play basketball. Rather than brushing off the idea, it was important to be creative and find other ways that David could participate in the basketball program. He was able to be a scorekeeper, assist the manager, and sit on the bench with the team. It was critical to motivate David and help him participate in an activity in which he was interested.

Encourage cooperative learning — If possible, it is better to choose an activity that is not based on competition, but rather encourages cooperation towards a common goal.

Be understandable — People who have disabilities are often more successful when involved in structured activities that have clear static rules, a well-defined beginning and end, a predictable or repetitive quality, and a clear visual representation of what to do.

Allow for social interaction — If the activity does not allow for a lot of social interaction, it is important to look for informal opportunities to socialize. For example, allow time for the person to arrive early or stay a little late so that they have the opportunity to socialize with the other participants. Another idea for creating social opportunities is car pooling with some of the other group members.

Be flexible — The activity should allow for adaptations to be made, if necessary, and allow the person to progress as he/she learns. For example, a person takes a pottery class and initially begins by making a pinch pot with assistance. Gradually, he/she needs less assistance and moves on to a more complicated project. With time and practice, he/she is able to mold clay on a pottery wheel independently.

Analyzing the community can be quite involved. However, your close attention to these steps and stages will clearly help the cultural shifting process. Careful observation of a culture paves the way for the next step in the process, which is identifying and recruiting a "gatekeeper." By studying the way that group members interact you can get a feeling for who the "key players" are and who may be helpful in welcoming a new member into that group.

"Not all leisure experiences in community settings need to be successful, but the privilege to achieve or fail is part of a learning process that for too long has been denied individuals with disabilities."

~ Stuart Schleien & M. Tipton Ray

Chapter Five
Finding the Gatekeeper

"Friendship is just like jazz...It's tough to define, but you know it when you hear it."

~ Miles Davis

Find and Engage the Gatekeeper

Every community has members who serve as gatekeepers.

A Gatekeeper: Someone who is already accepted and included in the culture (indigenous) and has some formal or informal influence within the culture.

That is, the gatekeeper has authority and influence with the members but may not have official authority for the group. When you think about it, often the most influential person in a community is not the official leader, but one of the regular members who commands respect. Coming to know who these persons are is an important step in building community.

Beyond this, it is important to know that gatekeepers can either be positive (supportive) or negative (resistant) in response to new things. The positive gatekeeper tends to be more accepting, open, and willing to take risks. The negative gatekeeper, on the other hand, is often more cautious and can be closed-minded. This positive or negative influence can be widespread. We all know people in our communities who are always positive and upbeat about life. They smile a lot and seem to always find the good in things. Conversely, we also know people who usually see the bad in life. These folks never seem to have a good day, and when you ask them how they are, you get an earful of woes.

When we think about gatekeepers in community, some psychologists suggest that we can easily apply the classic bell-shaped curve in which approximately 20 to 25% of people in the community would have the propensity to be positive or upbeat, with another 30 to 35% on the opposite end of the scale being negative. The remaining people, *who represent the majority of the community members*, are often neutral or unsure and could be swayed either way, depending on the influence and energy of dominant gatekeepers.

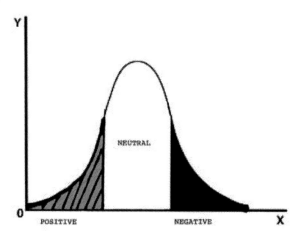

When the neutral members of a community get swayed either positively or negatively, we call this a "cultural shift." This is when a critical mass of the community begins to behave in a particular way. As stated earlier, gatekeepers can be formally elected or selected leaders (formal), or they might be one of the members who everyone can count on to get things done (informal). Think about the many gatekeepers you have had in your life as you have made your way into community. As we reflect on this, we can easily identify the people who immediately accepted us when we joined a new group. Additionally, we can remember those people who were not so nice to us.

When we were kids, we called those that accepted us "new friends" and those that were mean to us "bullies."

Now consider the clubs you have joined over the years or the times you moved to a new place, taken a new job, or went to a gathering for the first time. No matter where or when, we are convinced that a gatekeeper played a role in helping you get into the group. If this didn't happen, you probably left the gathering or bailed out of the party. Quite simply, we don't stay in communities where we are not welcomed. In this context, your gatekeepers are the people who embraced and welcomed you into the new venue. In fact, it is rare for anyone to get into a culture without the assistance of a gatekeeper. To this extent, gatekeepers, especially positive gatekeepers, are critical to culture because they help to bring new ideas into the community. When they do this, the new person introduced by the gatekeeper causes the existing members of the culture to define or redefine their position on the matter. This addition and redefinition of the culture is what leads to cultural growth.

The Positive Gatekeeper

Anthropologists have spent a good bit of time thinking about positive gatekeepers as they are vital to community growth. Some of the things we know about positive gatekeepers are:

- They tend to be optimistic people. They genuinely like people and look for the good in everyone they meet.
- They are social risk takers. They reach out to the underdog and are willing to take cultural flack if need be.
- They are open to new ideas and are curious and interested in why, how, and why not.
- They tend to be younger people and are not set in their ways.
- More often than not, they tend to be women. Men are usually more conservative and become more easily set in their ways.
- They are highly social and tend to be good mixers.
- They tend to have respect and influence in their community.
- They tend to be more creative and flexible.

If you want to bring a shift in cultural perspective, the endorsement and support of a gatekeeper is absolutely essential. The ability to identify and ask the gatekeeper for assistance without being perceived as attempting to meddle or influence is a true art in changing culture.

As you can see, finding the right gatekeeper is an essential part of getting a person who may be seen as different accepted into a new setting. If we can find a gatekeeper who has past experience with disability, or is sensitive to disability issues, he/she may be more apt to introduce the new person to their culture. Another point of connection may be that if the gatekeeper initially had a difficult time becoming a part of the group, then he/she may be more apt to sponsor a newcomer to make things easier for the new person. Similarly, people who perceive themselves to be more open-minded may have a greater willingness to accept differences and welcome someone new attempting to join the culture. Usually, positive gatekeepers are associated with emotional intelligence. This is the capacity to understand and tap into emotions in social relationships.

Think about your own personality. Are you a positive gatekeeper? Appendix D is an exercise entitled "Are You a Positive Gatekeeper?" Use the exercise to find out how open you are to new ideas. Thinking about the questions in this exercise might also help you to identify the positive gatekeepers that you already know. If so, can you use them as a resource in the process of helping a new person become an accepted member of your community?

The Gatekeeper

Gatekeepers come in many forms. They could be a child, program director, coach, volunteer, support person, community member, or parent. The ideal gatekeeper for children is another child within the group who will facilitate the new child's acceptance. If you are a parent of a child with a disability, you already know that this ideal does not always occur. Often, because of a fear of being rejected by their peers or because of a lack of knowledge about disability, children are reluctant to befriend a child who is seen as different. If this is the case, it is sometimes necessary to use an adult or older child to facilitate peer acceptance. The adult can be another parent, a volunteer, or a support person.

When a gatekeeper is an adult and not a group member, it is important to keep the following in mind:

If necessary:
- They should assist the coach or group leader.
- They should participate in the group activities.
- They should initiate activities that promote involvement of the child with a disability.
- They should physically assist with the activity.
- They should provide physical and verbal cues.

Always:
- They should get to know the other children in the group and serve as a link to the child with a disability.
- They should take advantage of unstructured time as an opportunity for socialization.

- They should have knowledge of and enjoy the activity.
- They should be willing to get to know the child with a disability.
- They should be creative in attracting other children to interact with the child with a disability.
- They should be able to help the child in acquiring skills.
- They should be able to teach the other children how to communicate with the child with a disability.
- They should minimize distractions by treating the child the same as all the other children.
- Most importantly, the gatekeeper/support person should know when to **back off** and allow natural social interactions to occur. It is important to maintain a continued awareness of how the child is participating in the activity and in what types of social interactions he/she is involved.
- The adult support person should try to encourage and support relationships that may lead to finding a natural gatekeeper within the group.

Recruiting the Gatekeeper

When joining a new group, recruiting a gatekeeper is not always an easy task. It can take a considerable amount of time and sensitivity. There is no definitive answer for how to facilitate friendships and encourage a reluctant gatekeeper.

"The ability to identify and then ask the gatekeeper for assistance is a true art in cultural change".

~Al Condeluci, 2002

Consider the following three strategies that might be useful when trying to identify and recruit a gatekeeper:

- Set goals that promote cooperation and encourage community members to support and assist one another rather than competing against one another. An example of this type of activity would be an after-school group working together to plan a party or a festival. This type of activity promotes social interaction and encourages the participants to work together in order to accomplish a common goal.
- Encourage another member of the group to assist the person with a disability in acquiring a skill. This is a helpful technique when trying to enlist a reluctant gatekeeper. Creating an opportunity for a gatekeeper to get to

know the person with a disability one-on-one may make the gatekeeper more eager to support that person within the group. One caution is to avoid the gatekeeper as seeing his/her role as a helper and not as a friend. (Schlien, 1997)
- Study the interactions between group members and restructure the group to promote positive social interactions. This means when you **observe** a group, take note of who the key players (the people with the most influence) are within that group. Also, observe the cliques that have formed within the group and which group members are being ignored. Then think about how you can **restructure** the group to break up cliques and promote interactions between the key players and the members of the group who have been rejected (Schlien, 1997).

These strategies are starting points that can help a child or adult with special needs find a connection within a group. This step in the process of cultural shifting will call for you to be creative. The important thing to remember is that if one strategy does not seem to be working, step back and consider trying something new.

Toward Friendships

A discussion on community inclusion without a discussion on friendship would be incomplete. Friendship and recreation are irrevocably intertwined; friendship enhances the recreation experience because it is made better by sharing it with a friend. Recreation activities provide opportunities to meet new people in situations in which differences in abilities are often minimized in favor of play, enjoyment and camaraderie. *Friendships typically grow and develop through shared recreation experiences.*

People with disabilities often have unique barriers that prevent them from developing and maintaining friendships. These barriers, however, are not insurmountable limitations that must preclude friendship development. Rather, these barriers should serve to challenge the creative teacher, family member, or recreation programmer to incorporate strategies for promoting friendship within the context of community recreation.

No matter what one's age may be, friendship plays an important role. When one has no friends, life spans are significantly reduced. Some experts have deemed friendship so essential that it has been called not an expendable luxury, but a necessity to life itself (Amado, 1993; Lynch, 1997).

Researchers have noted that even though people with disabilities may have opportunities to interact with peers, their actual social networks of friends and intimate relationships are substantially smaller than are the social networks of people without disabilities (Abery & Fahnestock, 1994; Vandercook, York, and Forest, 1989). Most of their relationships typically are limited to family members, acquaintances with disabilities, and people who are paid to interact with them. If you have created a sociogram on the individual for whom you are reading *Together is Better,* you may have realized this to be the case in his/her life.

Barriers to friendship appear to be a combination of individual social limitations as well as negative attitudes associated with disabilities. Consequently, an individual's abilities are often overlooked. There is no major strategy that will guarantee friendships for all people. Therefore, approaches to promoting friendships should be individualized to best meet the person's needs.

Some of the ways to encourage/facilitate friendships are:

- Groups can be restructured to promote positive interactions among members. This works best when a large group is broken down into smaller subgroups.
- Gather a small group of individuals who know the person with a disability. Perhaps you can elect a few people from the person's covenancy and friendship zones on his/her sociogram. These may be peers, service providers, family members, teachers, etc. Have these people identify the strengths and skills of the person with a disability. Identifying these qualities will serve as a starting point for forming friendships.
- Social awkwardness and uncomfortable feelings occur when there is a wide age range. It is best (especially when working with children) to group individuals together according to their age. This helps to promote ongoing friendships.
- Identify a person's interests and passions, such as sports, music, art, etc.

Family, school personnel, and community recreation staff all play a role in encouraging the growth of friendships between individuals with and without disabilities. How can this be done?

What families can do:
- Make friendship development a family priority — become acquainted with other families through school, church, community functions, or local sporting events.

- Schedule children's time together — families can request each other's phone numbers and addresses and take the initiative to call other parents.
- Learn about the individual needs of the child — to feel comfortable assuming responsibility for a child with special needs in their home, parents of children without disabilities need to learn about the child. For example, more information might be needed on mobility, communication, managing inappropriate behaviors, or personal care issues.
- Encourage positive social interaction skills — look for cooperative play and teach friendship skills.
- Learn about community resources — families need to explore their communities. Are there recreation centers, scouts, YMCA/YWCA, parks?

What schools can do:
- Provide opportunities for families to get together — sponsor open houses, PTA meetings, class trips, etc.
- Offer disability awareness training to all parents and teachers
- Encourage children to work in group settings and have teachers supervise and make suggestions

What staff at Community Centers can do:
- Include all children
- Educate staff and have available support if needed
- Ensure accessibility
- Coordinate after-school/weekend activities
- Encourage all children to be involved to their fullest potential
- Provide an environment that is conducive to friendship development

Friendship is more than acquaintance. Being a friend is different from being a volunteer. It usually develops out of mutual interests and common goals. Real friendship possesses virtues, loyalty, and trust, and offers help in time of need. Friendship does not just bring you happiness, it makes you a better person. It also can promote positive changes in the behavior of people with disabilities. Above all, friendship encourages a sense of belonging and connectedness.

> *"Friendship makes prosperity more shining and lessens adversity by dividing it and sharing it."*
>
> *~ Cicero*

Conclusion
Journeying Forward

"Never doubt that a small group of thoughtful, committed citizens can change the world. Indeed it is the only thing that ever has."

~Margaret Mead

Journeying Forward

The challenge of a full and inclusive community for all people is a never-ending goal. Not only are there architectural barriers and severe limitations in the physical capacity of community to be more inviting, but there are also the attitudinal perspectives of community members that can be even more challenging.

For years, typical community members have perceived people with disabilities as infirm, sick, or incapable of full participation. These attitudes have run long and deep. Add to this the historical institutionalization that has encased disability, and you have formidable obstacles to the goal of mainstreaming and inclusion.

Even though advocates have chipped away at the architectural and attitudinal barriers, we still have the continued exclusion of people with disabilities. This exclusion has manifested in special and separate programs that are still all-encompassing. Today when a family is told that their child has a disability, the march of separate and specialized programs begins. Offset programs, support groups, and specialized services become the norm, and families begin to see these specialized resources as the answer. Combine this with the systematic reality that specialized agencies see it as their job to address the needs of their constituents — and more programs are produced. Subsequently, a dualistic world is created. One is for people with disabilities; the other is for the rest of us.

This is not to say that specialized programs are bad or unnecessary. Some, maybe most, are good efforts. The reality, however, is that for every hour an individual spends in a specialized program, it is one less hour that the individual is within his or her own natural community. And perhaps even more disheartening, it is one less hour that the *community* has the opportunity to interact with the individual. Because of this lack of interaction, this reality teaches the community a powerful lesson – that the person with a disability is better off in a specialized place.

The basic crux of this manual is the exact opposite.

It is our belief that all people have more in common than they are different. We also know that all people have some basic differences, but it is our similarities that begin to bond us with others and lead to the start of social capital. We feel strongly that when differences flow in a sea of commonality, all the boats rise.

It has been the intention of this manual to challenge the assumptions of separation. We know that there may be times when some people need to be separated, but these times should be minimal, for **when we are together, we are better.**

In a sense, we have become prisoners of our own success. As we have focused to better understand disabilities, we have created new worlds for those with disabilities. These worlds have harnessed many people and have denied our generic communities the riches of difference.

Through our experiences at UCP Pittsburgh in working with adults with disabilities and through our UCP Kids program, we have come to know several things:

- We know that the earlier we start building full and inclusive communities, the long-term implications for people with disabilities will be entirely different than they are today. But while we know that "the sooner, the better," we also know that it is never too late. Adults with disabilities can have rewarding experiences and full lives. Children with disabilities can flourish and form true friendships.
- We know that the social capital we find in our relationships is good for us. The more we have, the happier we seem to be. We know that people with more social capital have less sick days and live longer, more rewarding lives.
- We know that building social capital is predicated not on differences but on similarities. The more we have in common with other people, the easier it is for us to bridge with them and thus develop the bonding relationships that enhance life and that challenge us to grow.

Together is Better *is an effort to intentionally use this information in the challenge of full* inclusion.

Now it is time for you to set this manual aside. For many, you have already developed your social capital. You know in your heart that the only way others are going to really experience social capital is to find the opportunity to connect with new people. So let's get to it.

Every journey starts with the first step. Best of luck on the path!

> *"When I think of why my daughter should be included in education and recreation activities in our community, many things come to mind. I know that she will have fun and is motivated by learning from other children. I also feel it is important that she develop 'broad shoulders' due to the initial reactions to her disability, which is a skill that will benefit her as an adult. Most importantly, through these experiences, my daughter will be making vital connections within the community by meeting the children who may someday be her neighbors, employers or fellow employees. Becoming linked as children will broaden future opportunities for both my daughter and children without disabilities by allowing their tolerance of differences to grow and fear to fade away."*
>
> *~ Robin Foley*

Appendix A

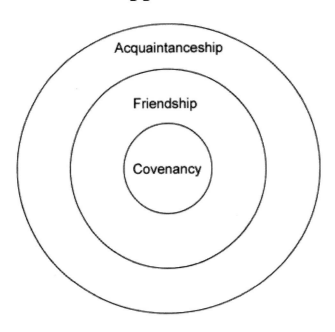

1. The Covenancy Zone

In the space below, we want you to identify the first group in the individual's sociogram, the people to whom he/she is closest. Please write down the names of all those people in his/her life with whom deep relationships exist. These are the people that he/she spends the most amount of time with and has the most reciprocity.

_____
_____
_____
_____
_____
_____
_____
_____

Together is Better

2. The Friendship Zone

These are the people with whom the individual shares common interests and frequently engages in activities. In this group would be those people with whom he/she goes to dinner, bowls, plays bridge, goes to the theatre, or whatever the mutual interest may be. These are his/her friends who are not merely casual friends, but friendships that manifest themselves, friends with whom he/she chooses to spend quality time. Reflect a bit on this and then write their names below. Remember, these are people who often participate in activities with the individual but who are *not* included in his/her covenancy zone.

_____
_____
_____
_____
_____
_____
_____
_____
_____
_____
_____
_____
_____
_____
_____
_____
_____
_____
_____
_____
_____
_____
_____
_____

3. The Acquaintanceship Zone

In the space below, we want you to identify all of the people who the individual knows and even sees regularly, but with whom he/she does not purposely engage in activities. These are acquaintances he/she has at work, school, church, and in the community. He/she knows these people, but doesn't actually exchange any real time with them. In fact, this category often includes people from whom he/she purchases products or services in the course of everyday life. These people include beauticians or barbers, mechanics, medical personnel, or butchers. They might all be people he/she knows, but never actually engages other than to buy what they offer. He/she sees these people on a regular basis and knows them, but does not really participate in activities with them. As you think about this list, name only the people that *currently* fit into this category in his/her life. List them below:

Appendix B

Kids Interest Profile

What are your child's favorite things to do? / What makes your child happy?

- ☐ Foods
- ☐ Games
- ☐ Going places
- ☐ Music/Sounds
- ☐ Socializing
- ☐ Reading
- ☐ Being alone
- ☐ Animals
- ☐ Tactile (touch)
- ☐ Being sung to
- ☐ TV shows
- ☐ Other

What are a few of your child's best qualities?

_____

_____

_____

What motivates your child?

- ☐ Playtime
- ☐ Music
- ☐ Food
- ☐ Toys
- ☐ Person
- ☐ TV
- ☐ Money
- ☐ Animals
- ☐ Privileges
- ☐ Other

What calms your child?

- ☐ Holding
- ☐ Being talked to
- ☐ Playing
- ☐ Rocking
- ☐ Music
- ☐ Being sung to
- ☐ Laughter
- ☐ Other

What does your child dislike?

- ☐ Noise
- ☐ Rushing
- ☐ Eating
- ☐ Foods
- ☐ Smells
- ☐ Rules
- ☐ Tastes
- ☐ Being alone
- ☐ Crowds
- ☐ Tactile
- ☐ Other

What does your child use as a coping mechanism?
- ☐ Safe person
- ☐ Safe place
- ☐ Oral stimulation
- ☐ Body movement
- ☐ Familiar object
- ☐ Withdrawal
- ☐ Becomes hyper
- ☐ Other

What does your child fear?
- ☐ Sounds
- ☐ Crowds
- ☐ Movement
- ☐ Adults
- ☐ Other children
- ☐ Falling
- ☐ Animals
- ☐ Water
- ☐ Darkness

Group and Activity Participation

1) What types of groups does your family belong to (church, recreational groups, etc.)?

_____

_____

_____

_____

_____

a) How often does your family participate in these groups?

_____

_____

_____

_____

b) How comfortable do you feel when you participate in these groups?
☐ Very Comfortable ☐ Somewhat Comfortable ☐ Uncomfortable ☐ Very Uncomfortable

c) What if any barriers have you encountered when participating in these groups?

_____

_____

2) What types of groups does your child belong to (church, school, sports, scouts, etc.)?

   a) How often does he/she participate in these groups?

   b) How comfortable does your child feel when participating in these groups?
   ☐ Very Comfortable ☐ Somewhat Comfortable ☐ Uncomfortable ☐ Very Uncomfortable

   c) What if any barriers has your child encountered when participating in these groups?

3) What activities does your family participate in with other families or relatives (outings, reunions, vacations, etc.)?

a) How often does your family participate in these activities?

_____

_____

_____

b) How comfortable do you feel when participating in these activities?
☐ Very Comfortable ☐ Somewhat Comfortable ☐ Uncomfortable ☐ Very Uncomfortable

c) What if any barriers have you encountered when participating in these activities?

_____

_____

_____

_____

4) What neighborhood/community events (block parties, pot luck dinners, parades, picnics/ cookouts, etc.) does your family attend?

_____

_____

_____

a) How often does your family attend these events?

_____

_____

_____

b) How comfortable do you feel when you attend these events?
☐ Very Comfortable ☐ Somewhat Comfortable ☐ Uncomfortable ☐ Very Uncomfortable

c) What if any barriers have you encountered when participating in these activities?

_____
_____
_____

5) What neighborhood/community events (block parties, pot luck dinners, parades, picnics/cookouts, etc.) does your family attend?

_____
_____
_____
_____

a) How often does your family attend these events?

_____
_____
_____
_____

b) How comfortable do you feel when you attend these events?
☐ Very Comfortable ☐ Somewhat Comfortable ☐ Uncomfortable ☐ Very Uncomfortable

c) What if any barriers have you encountered when attending these events?

_____
_____
_____
_____

6) What events does your child's school have?

_____
_____
_____
_____

a) How often does your child or family attend these events?

_____
_____
_____
_____

b) How comfortable do you feel when you attend these events?
☐ Very Comfortable ☐ Somewhat Comfortable ☐ Uncomfortable ☐ Very Uncomfortable

c) What if any barriers have you or your child encountered when attending these events?

_____
_____
_____

Relationships

2) On a scale of 0 to 10 with 10 being excellent, how would you rate the quality of the relationships your child has with:

a) Children in your neighborhood? _____

b) Students in his/her school? _____

c) His/her relatives (cousins, aunts, uncles, grandparents, etc.) _____

Comments on relationships rated above:

_____
_____
_____

List any activities that your child would like to participate in that he/she is not involved in currently:

_____
_____
_____

Is there anything that someone who works with your child should know about their health?

_____
_____
_____

Is there anything that someone who works with your child should know about the way your child communicates?

_____
_____
_____

What do you hope being involved in the UCP Kids project will do for your child/your family?

_____
_____
_____

Interest Profile created by the staff of UCP Kids in partnership with the Office of Child Development at the University of Pittsburgh

Appendix C

Activity Analysis

Steps of the Activity + - **Adaptations/Modifications**

Together is Better

Appendix C

Activity Analysis

Steps of the Activity + - **Adaptations/Modifications**

Appendix D

Are you a Positive Gatekeeper?

Circle either **a** or **b** to indicate how you usually are in these situations:

1. If someone disagrees with me in a meeting or a group, I
    a. immediately back down
    b. explain my position further
2. When I have an idea for a project, I
    a. typically take a great deal of time to start it
    b. get going on it fairly quickly
3. If my boss or group leader tells me to do something that I think is wrong, I
    a. do it anyway, telling myself he or she is the boss
    b. ask for clarification and explain my position
4. When a complicated problem arises, I usually tell myself
    a. I can take care of it
    b. I will not be able to solve it
5. When I am around people of higher authority, I often
    a. feel intimidated and defer to them
    b. enjoy meeting important people
6. As I awake in the morning, I usually feel
    a. alert and ready to conquer almost anything
    b. tired and have a hard time getting myself motivated
7. During an argument, I
    a. criticize myself on what I am doing or thinking
    b. try to listen to the other side and see if we have any points of agreement
8. When I meet new people, I
    a. always wonder what they are really up to
    b. try to learn what they are about and give them the benefit of the doubt until they prove otherwise
9. During the day, I often
    a. criticize myself on what I am doing or thinking
    b. think positive thoughts about myself

10. When someone else does a great job, I
    a. find myself picking apart that person and looking for faults
    b. often give a sincere compliment
11. When I am working in a group, I try to
    a. do a better job than the others
    b. help the group function more effectively
12. If someone pays me a compliment, I typically
    a. try not to appear boastful and downplay the compliment
    b. respond with a positive "thank you" or similar response
13. I like to be around people who
    a. challenge me and make me question what I do
    b. give me respect
14. In love relationships, I prefer the other person to
    a. have his/her own selected interests
    b. do pretty much what I do
15. During a crisis, I try to
    a. resolve the problem
    b. find someone to blame
16. After seeing a movie with my friends, I
    a. wait to see what they say before I decide whether I liked it
    b. am ready to talk about my reactions right away
17. When work deadlines are approaching, I typically
    a. get flustered and worry about completion
    b. buckle down and work until the job is done
18. If a job comes up I am interested in, I
    a. go for it and apply
    b. tell myself that I am not qualified enough
19. When someone treats me unkindly or unfairly, I
    a. try to rectify the situation
    b. tell other people about the injustice
20. If a difficult conflict situation or problem arises, I
    a. try not to think about it hoping it will resolve itself
    b. look for various options and may ask others for advice before

Analysis of Scoring

16-20 You are a positive gatekeeper and generally make the most of opportunities. When others tell you something cannot be done, you may take this as a challenge and do it anyway. You see the world as your oyster with many pearls to harvest.

11-15 You try hard, but sometimes your negative attitude prevents you from getting involved in productive projects. Many times you take responsibility, but there are situations where you look to others to take care of problems.

0-10 You complain too much and are usually focused on the "worst case scenario." To you, the world is controlled by fate and no matter what you do it seems to get you nowhere, so you let other people develop opportunities. You need to start seeing the positive qualities in yourself and in others and see yourself as the "master of your fate."

Scoring:
Score one point for each of the following circled:

1b, 2b, 3b, 4a, 5b, 6a, 7b, 8b, 9b, 10b, 11b, 12b, 13a, 14a, 15a, 16b, 17b, 18a, 19a, 20b

Resources

Websites

www.aaasp.org
American Association of Adapted Sports Programs

www.tash.org
Supports the inclusion and full participation of children and adults with disabilities in all aspects of communities

www.ncpad.org
The National Center on Physical Activity and Disability

www.new-horizons.org
New Horizons Un-Limited
Community and recreation resources, including specialized adaptive sports equipment companies

www.ucppittsburgh.org
United Cerebral Palsy
Promotes inclusion of children and adults with disabilities into community

Books

Condeluci, A. (2004). *Advocacy for Change: A Manual for Action.* Alexandria, VA: ANCOR.

Condeluci, A. (2002). *Cultural Shifting: Community Leadership and Change.* St. Augustine, FL: Training Resouce Network, Inc.

Condeluci, A. (1999). *The Essence of Interdependence.* Baco Raton, FL: CRC Press.

Condeluci, A. (1996). *Beyond Difference.* Delray Beach, FL: St.Lucie Press.

Condeluci, A. (1995). *Interdependence: The Route to Community.* Baco Raton, FL: CRC Press.

Moon, S. (1994). *Making School and Community Recreation Fun for Everyone: Places and Ways to Integrate.* Baltimore, MD: Paul H. Brookes Publishing Co.

Wolfberg, P. (2003). *Peer Play and the Autism Spectrum: The art of guiding children's socialization and imagination.* Shawnee Mission, KS: Autism Asperger Publishing Co.

Bibliography

The Anatomy of Friendships." *Tash Connections.* January/February 2004.

American Association for Active Lifestyles and Fitness. www.aaasp.org

Bellah, Robert. (1985). *Habits of the Heart.* New York: Harper and Row.

"Building Community Resources." *Exceptional Parent.* July 1995.

Condeluci, A. (2002). *Cultural Shifting: Community Leadership and Change.* St. Augustine, FL: Training Resource Network, Inc.

Coyne, P; Nyberg, C; Vandenburg, M. (1999). *Developing Leisure Time Skills for Persons with Autism: A Practical Approach for Home, School and Community.* Arlington: Future Horizons Inc.

Dunst, C; Herter, S; Shields, H; & Bennis, L (in press). Mapping community-based natural learning opportunities. *Young Exceptional Children.*

Gladwell, M. (2000). *The Tipping Point.* New York: Little, Brown and Co.

"A Guide to Knowing Your Community." *Center on Human Policy.* Winter 1990.

Putnam, R. (2000). *Bowling Alone.* New York: Simon and Schuster.

Schlein, Stewart. *Community Recreation and People with Disabilities: Strategies for Inclusion.*

"Social Skills on the Playground." *Autism Digest Magazine.* March – April 2004.